Recovery Now!

Kick-starting Your Health

By Andrew Gillies

Dedicated to Margaret and John

Disclaimer

Information found in this book is not a substitute for medical advice. Always consult a professional healthcare provider before beginning any new treatment. It is the responsibility of the reader to research the accuracy and usefulness of all information found at this site.

The author assumes no responsibility or liability for any consequence resulting directly or indirectly for any action or inaction you take based on or made in reliance on the information, services, or material on or linked to this book. All information provided in this book is for informational purposes only.

This book contains links to sites and services. In no event shall the author be held responsible or liable, directly or indirectly, for any damage or loss caused or alleged to be caused by, or in connection with the use of or reliance on any such content, goods, or services available on or through any site or resource.

Introduction

This isn't a long book, I feel it would be counter-productive for any reader to spend a lot of time reading this, and ideally I feel it would probably be best read in as few sittings as possible. I am neither a doctor nor do I claim to be anywhere near being an authority when it comes to the sciences, so this is not a technical book nor a complicated book. There may be some new ways of looking at things to consider, but they are not difficult to understand. What this book aims to do is to give you hope, to give you a new way of understanding health and illness, and to those that it pertains to, it will give you a new way to proceed.. It's a kick start book, designed to facilitate a change in your focus, your state of mind and your state of health.

I wouldn't claim to be the embodiment of health myself, my back aches sometimes, I get pains here and there, pretty regular stuff. All of which begs the question.....in what way am I qualified to talk on this subject? Well, my Mum was diagnosed with a 'terminal' illness, which turned out to be 'terminal' over a period of about fourteen years (the word 'terminal' is so flawed and outdated these days, in one way, we are 'terminal' from the moment we are born!). She outlived her prognosis by a long way, and for a while, it genuinely seemed as if she could, and would, make a recovery. She didn't, though there was a quality of peace to her passing, a sense that it was the right time for her, and this is important.

I learned enough during my time supporting her over the whole period (and in the last two and a half years I was with her pretty much all day every day), to know that recovery from serious illness is very much possible these days, even when the diagnosis says that death is inevitable. I didn't just learn this through being with my Mum, I learned this through hours and hours of research into the nature of health and illness, through studying those that have recovered from so called terminal illness, and through understanding the process by which normal people achieve goals and realize their dreams.

None of what I learned guarantees recovery. Death happens. Sometime people are ready for death, it is the most appropriate step for them, the soul is ready to transition. Quite honestly, sometimes death is a welcome thing, and if this is our truth, then allowing ourselves to know that is important. Sometimes the most valuable lesson in the face of death is finding acceptance, and enjoying the last chapter of our lives as much as possible. This doesn't even necessarily apply to the elders of our society, sometimes a twenty year old can sense the truth that it is their time, that they did whatever they needed to do here, and that is perfect.

For many though, this doesn't necessarily apply. At the physical human level, we may feel that we have much to offer, that we're not done, that there is still an adventure to be found in the world. At a bare minimum, we are at a stage of evolution at which it would be very nice to feel like we have a choice! That the potential IS there to recover despite an extremely negative prognosis.

So this book is written specifically for those that sense that this doesn't have to be their time, but on the other hand just aren't quite sure WHAT to do. It's for those that don't want to wait for the medical institutions and industry to turn up a cure. It's for those that want to, and are willing, to take action. You may not be sure if that is you or not, and that's okay, sometimes old fashioned societal conditioning can get in the way of our true intentions and desires and muddy the waters. This book will help you work through that too.

Alternatively, you might be someone reading the book on behalf of a loved one that is sick….three years ago….I might well have been reading this too. Please know that while the path another soul chooses is entirely theirs, that you are not separate from that path, that we are each co-participators in Life, and that if you feel positive about what is being said in this book, then that is doing your loved one good, and anyone else that also has that illness.

Hope

The first thing to do is get on the internet and start exploring recovery stories. It doesn't matter if you have Crohn's, M.S, Parkinson's, Cancer or any other illness, get online and find out what people around the world are doing to address your issue and related issues. There is likely to be a support group and forum dedicated to your specific condition, and although these can be useful, some forums can also be fairly negative, and that's not the fault of the forum or the people on it, it is what it is.

People are likely to give you sympathy and empathy on a forum and that's nice n' all, but those in particular you want to look for are the ones that are getting definite positive results from whatever they are doing. When you find them, avoid telling yourself the story 'That wouldn't work for me' or 'I couldn't do that' or perhaps 'Oh, it's working for them now, but it will stop working for them at some point'. When things aren't going well, it's normal to feel slightly envious or jealous of those that are getting results, but put those feelings to one side and take heart from the fact that there are people getting good results. Really open to up the possibility that other people are doing something that's making a difference, and could make a difference to you too.

Specialist forums are just the tip of the iceberg though, there are people out there that want to share what worked for them and are telling their story on YouTube, or on their own website. Google wisely. ''Recovery from Parkinson's'' is a good example, or *'Full* recovery' might be an even better search. You will find stories of people recovering from most illnesses, including Alzheimer's, Parkinson's, Fibromyalgia, M.S, M.E,

ALS, Cancer of all different kinds. I have also seen stories of people that have recovered from Aids. It's a definite bonus if you can find people that have recovered from your illness, but just reading and listening to people talk about how they changed their situation, whatever it was, is inspiring, educational and good to hear. I'm not going to say I researched every story to see if it was actually true, but even if some of them are made up (and I don't believe many are), there is still a huge amount of positivity on the web.

These are largely people that did something different, that chose not to ONLY go the allopathic route. To be clear, I believe the allopathic route has a huge amount to offer, but it's not the only route, perhaps also not the best route in certain situations.

The allopathic route has traditionally dealt with the mechanics of the human body, and this is useful and has its place, but it basically starts from the assumption that the problem has happened TO the individual. Many that get interesting results outside of the allopathic route (and even within it) start from the assumption that the individual is actively involved to at least some extent with the creation of his/her state of health/illness. From a more 'holistic' perspective, instead of just looking at an illness (and the body) as something to be mechanically fixed, we can look at the individual him/herself i.e. what is going on in the individual's experience, what are the individual's *sensitivities,* what is the psychology of the individual, and also what might the individual be getting out OF the illness. This isn't remotely a suggestion to go into deep therapy for the next year, it's an invitation to assume that you are playing some kind of participatory role in the creation of the illness, rather than standing back from it as if it some alien entity that has invaded the body.

Of course, most doctors wouldn't likely deny that smoking is bad for health or that too much stress can have a negative effect on the body, they are happy to look at causes of sickness, and this is useful, but what they don't tend to look at is the *purpose* of the illness, they don't look at the relationship *between* the individual and the illness.

So when you are reading and listening to how other people have recovered (or are recovering), obviously look at what practical alternative steps they took, but also look at the way they mentally, emotionally and energetically addressed their situation. Look at their attitude, their approach, what they think and feel, what they focus upon, and what drives them.

In all cases I have seen, there is a congruent and authentic desire to be well. It feels right to them that they could and should be well. This isn't from a place of "I did nothing to deserve this horrible illness, so I should be well", it's from a place of recognizing that they have more to give in life, more to explore, more to experience. That it's not their time to transition.

Secondly, they are open to doing things differently. They haven't bought into the prognosis. They have gone against society. They have gone against the 'authority figure' that the medical institution presents itself as. There is a rebellious streak there. There is some belief in their own ability to find a way to be well. There is a willingness to work WITH their body, rather than fight the body, and an understanding that whatever the organism is doing is for a reason, and it is always doing its best. It's not the case that the body has 'failed' you, it's not the case the body has 'turned on' its owner, it's not the case that what's happening with the body has very little to do with you. Instead, it is understood that what is being created within the body can also be undone, and that something else can be created instead.

Sometimes the solution is very simple and doesn't require a lot more than being willing to do things differently, to try out a few 'crazy' things. For Cancer, there is (to name just a few examples) the Gerson Diet, the Dr Budwig diet, the protocel approach, Cesium therapy, plus Cannabis oil which is a remedy that gets great results for many people for many different illnesses. The 'zapper' is another example of an alternative approach that gets great results. Hydrogen Peroxide is another. Homeopathy can get negative publicity in the popular media but I have read some great success stories. The effect of coconut oil and turmeric has had some interesting feedback in relation to Alzheimer's. Herbs, supplements and flower remedies can also be perhaps surprisingly effective for some conditions. Then there is the power of guided imagery and visualization, which definitely should not be underestimated in its efficacy. In regard to autism, the wonderful book 'The Horse Boy' by Rupert Isaacson reveals that there is much that can be done.

What I have noticed is that it's not always the case that someone takes steps, gets results, and then is actually medically assessed to be 'cured' of the illness. What is important is that the illness becomes irrelevant to your life. If there are no symptoms of Parkinson's showing up in the body at all, then it really doesn't matter if it has been officially 'cured' or not! I have sometimes seen the allopathic institution say when someone reports that they have recovered from an illness, that they didn't have it to start with, or that they must have had a different illness to the one that was diagnosed, and that may be true in some cases, but really.....I think this is the institution feeling forced to defend itself.

This reminds me of my Mum, who told me more than once that one thing she found intimidating about the potential of getting well was the prospect of people believing that she had been lying about the illness in some way, or making it up! She certainly would have been happy to take a magic pill from the doctor for the illness, but one of her insecurities was that if she 'got well' through an alternative means, then people might wonder if she had been playing games for many years. In a way, she also didn't want to upset the doctors or make them look bad, there was a definite sense of obligation there to be unwell in the way that she was 'supposed' to. Such is the power though of established norms, which is why when we take an alternative route and get results, we are somewhat obliged to stand out from the crowd, which we may be a bit reticent about depending on our nature.

So, it is very important to find hope and to have hope, because hope gives us strength to get moving, and to take positive action in the face of seeming adversity. Genuinely, there really IS hope, and the gift of the world wide web can show you this beyond doubt. The planet isn't what it was thirty years ago when people from different nations and cultures weren't able to communicate with each other easily, these days the world is much more of a community, and a huge amount of information is shared. There are people out there that have recovered from the worst of prognoses, and many of them want to share what they learned.

Though to be clear, I'm not inviting you to have a sort of *passive* hope that 'a miracle cure will come along soon', this is a hope that is born out of the knowing that there is something YOU can do. You are neither powerless, nor a victim of a terrible affliction. You have an actual relationship with your body-mind, and together, you CAN create a state of health.

The Promise

This is a promise, the only promise I am willing to make in the book:

If you can imagine yourself to be well, if you can imagine a life of health and wellness for yourself, if you can imagine *freedom*, whatever that looks like for you, then you CAN get well.

If you can congruently feel how it would feel to be healthy and well, if you can clearly see the life you want without the illness, if you can clearly see what you want to do in a renewed and rejuvenated state of health, if you feel your future relationships from a place of being healthy and happy....then the potential is definitely there to be healthy and well.

****

Now, to be clear, I understand that envisioning and feeling yourself to be healthy and well, may not necessarily be an easy thing to do, so if you can't do it straight away, that's okay. It can take a bit of renewed hope, a bit of commitment and a bit of practice to do this. When illness and sickness has prevailed for a long time, and it's been tough, we have to find a way to get through it, and it can be damn hard. In enduring the hardship, sometimes we have to switch off the aspect of our mind that can clearly envision and dream in a positive way. When we are used to feeling bad, it can be genuinely hard to feel good! Plus, there can be a lot of emotional resistance to having the dream, in the sense that we don't want to dream about what we believe we can't have…it hurts! Plus, we might have a sense of not wanting to get our hopes up, only to be disappointed.

So I know there are valid reasons why it can be difficult to imagine ourselves to be healthy and well from a place of sickness, especially if it has been debilitating over a long period. Furthermore, when there has been a long term condition and we try to imagine wellness, we often naturally try to imagine who we were prior to the illness and the kind of life we were living back then. However, trying to imagine returning to that often doesn't quite work because we are also not quite the same person we were. The experience of being ill changes us (as all significant life experiences do), and there is no shame in that. In a way, it's MEANT to change us, it gives us a new perspective on life, it impacts on our priorities and values, and we have the potential to mature, learn and grow from these kinds of experiences. As much as we may miss our life prior to the illness, as a result of the change, it can be difficult to congruently and authentically imagine going back to our old life. We have to be willing to move forward rather than go back, and this can be a challenge if we get comfort from our memories.

Imagining a positive new life doesn't mean that we have to imagine a *radically* new life, a life that is a total departure from our old life, we may just return to our old routines with a new perspective on life, and a renewed sense of appreciation perhaps. It is important though to look forward in the most positive way we can. A good way is to ask ourselves what we would LOVE to do if we recovered. It might be walks in the park, going on vacation, going to parties, going to university. How would we celebrate our new life of health and wellness? Would we appreciate and love our family even more, would we go and do the thing we always said we were going to do, would we stop and smell the roses more, would we go and teach what we always wanted to teach?

There are so many different options here depending on the individual. Obviously age is going to be a factor! The dream doesn't have to be a BIG dream, it just has to be *congruent,* in other words, it has to be true for you. If you are a grandparent and can joyfully imagine watching your grand-children growing up, that's good enough!

Allowing yourself to imagine a healthy future can take a lot of courage, but the principles beneath this are sound and I am going to explain them in brief:

Basically, it doesn't make a significant difference to your brain whether you are imagining doing something, or actually doing that something. The brain doesn't distinguish between reality and imagination. For example, studies have amazingly shown that just imagining doing a physical workout can have an effect on the muscles of the body! In Dr David Hamilton's words, '''Neuroscience research shows that the same areas of the brain are activated regardless of whether a person does actual training or simulates it in their minds. And, incredibly, the amount of force produced by the muscles is directly proportional to the degree of activation of the brain area. In other words, the more you activate the brain through mental work, the stronger the muscle.''

And as the forward thinking and very interesting website www.inmindinbody.com says....

''Simply watching or listening to the description of a movement stimulates the respective muscles in your own body (Buccino et al. 2004, Porro et al., 2007 and Ertelt et al., 2007) as they activate neurons in the part of the brain controlling the muscle movement involved. This explains why we wince when we see someone else experiencing pain.

Porro et al. (2007) asked a group of individuals to train the little finger in their right hand, by repeatedly flexing it over a period of time. They asked a second group of individuals to merely watch the first group, and by the end of the study both groups and experienced an increase in the strength of their little finger, the first by 50% and the second by 32%. Additionally, the strength of the left hand little finger also increased in both groups, the first by 33% and the second by 30%.

In addition to this study, Ertelt et al. (2007) discovered regeneration in the brain maps of stroke patients after they had watched people repeat everyday actions, such as eating and drinking, as well as receiving their normal rehabilitation. These patients had improved much more greatly by the end of the study than patients who had not watched the actions.

Buccino et al. (2004) discovered that the area of the brain controlling hand movements was activated when volunteers listened to people talking about hand movements. The same was discovered for feet.

The brain is likened to a muscle, the more you use it the more powerful it becomes

In the same way as muscles, we can train and grow our brain, as it is also activated through imagining. Pascual-Leone et al. (1995) asked a group of individuals to perform a repeated five-finger sequence of notes on the piano. This was carried out for two hours a day for five consecutive days. A second group was asked to imagine playing and hearing the notes for the same period of time. The area of the brain which controls finger movement had grown to the same extent in both groups.

Muscles grow if we imagine using them

A study by Ranganathan et al. (2004) demonstrated an increase in muscular strength through imagined exercise. Participants undertook physical training over a period of weeks, with some imagining doing the same training instead. The training involved exercising participants little finger, with 15 contractions followed by a short rest period, repeated for 15 minutes. This was completed five days a week for five weeks. Both sets of participants gained muscular strength in their little finger; those who did the physical training by 53%, those imagining doing so by 35%."

****

This is a whole new way of understanding the body, the brain and our relationship to life itself, and for those that are interested, it's well worth exploring. Lisa Rankin, Dr Joe Dispenza, Lynne McTaggart and Dr Deepak Chopra are great authors and a search for them on amazon will reveal many others that are also doing very interesting work on this subject. They all also have many talks on YouTube that are well worth watching, they are inspiring, and will give you hope and encouragement. However, if it's not the kind of thing you are interested in understanding in depth, that's fine, it's not necessary as long as you are willing to take the basic points on board. Science has changed a lot in fifty years, and understanding even just a bit about this if you don't already is useful.

What is important for you to understand is that you can make your brain work for you. Actually you already are making it work for you, you just may not be aware of it. Crucially, in addition to the massive amount of jobs the brain carries out in relation to the body's overall functioning, it specifically follows our 'direction' and in that sense it is entirely neutral, just as any tool is. Specifically, what we focus upon, we get more of. The reason is, that our brain has to filter the incredible amount of information that exists in the universe, so it filters out all that does not relate to our interests and our beliefs, so that what we perceive therefore pertains specifically to what we already believe. In a sense, it's like an ongoing confirmation bias, in the sense that what we give attention is determined by our beliefs, which in turn will tend to reinforce our world view, unless and until something big enough disrupts it. This is why it can sometimes take an enormous amount of evidence to change a popular view of something.

So if we are focused on the impossibility of recovery, If we are focused upon how bad we feel and how rotten the illness is and how unfair life is….then the brain says...'oh okay, so you are interested in the impossibility of recovery, in feeling bad, and being sick'....and what we will perceive will reinforce that, for example what we will be primarily notice is people struggling with the illness, we will notice negative reports, we will notice things that either won't help us, or that we won't believe will help us.

On the other hand, we can condition ourselves to focus upon our desire and to where we want to go, to find value in our current situation, and to take the opportunities to feel good when we can. The brain gets the message and says 'oh okay, so you are interested in being well and feeling well'. Over a period of time, the brain adjusts (new neural pathways open) and it becomes very easy and natural to be a positive leaning person. We may not instantly recover, but as a result of this, we will, without a doubt, find ourselves moving in a different direction. Different things will catch our eye, new people that can help us will pop up, new opportunities will present themselves, and new doors will open. This can all happen VERY quickly. If you are reading this book, then that's already a good sign of where your focus is placed.

The 'directional' nature of our brain can be seen to apply in all walks of life: anyone that has large amounts of money, great sportspeople, inventors, chefs, musicians...even healers....whether they know it or not, they all believe in their potential, and the potential of Life itself. As such, they are consistently more focused on where they are going, than what they can't have. They are more focused on their desire, than they are their limitations. Of course, there are times to recognize what isn't working within that, but their overall mind set and frame of reference leans towards 'can do' than 'can't do', in fact, it leans towards 'WILL do' rather than 'won't do'.

A great example that relates to what we are talking about here, is actually the well known placebo effect, though it is fascinating that it is often given a negative connotation, as if it is a bad thing, getting in the way of proper medicine. In actuality, the placebo effect reveals much about the relationship between mind, body and brain. If we think we are going to get well, then that does have an effect on us. We can USE the placebo effect deliberately to help us to get well. I think it's true to say that in the old days it was seen as somewhat 'weak-minded' to allow the mind to be 'swayed' in this way, we have to get over that stigma and recognize that there is something profound going on here. Many of us were taught that 'seeing is believing', but it's beginning to look like there is equal validity to the idea that 'believing is seeing' i.e. when we believe it, we will see it.

If you can find it (and I'm sure you can these days), watch Derren Brown's one off special entitled 'Fear and Faith', which was a study of the placebo effect. He worked with a few subjects that had long term debilitating fears/phobias, a group of smokers, and some people with allergy issues and eczema. He created a fake drug, fostered a trust in the drug within the subjects, and using his myriad of skills, invited them to give themselves permission to act as if their problems didn't exist anymore. The results were amazing. Aside from one of the subjects (and Derren worked with her further at the end to very successfully facilitate a change), they each overcame their issues. It was overall a great example of how the somewhat stigmatized idea of the placebo effect can be explored and used in a very positive way. Creating a strong sense of belief is key and you can build that sense of belief really quite easily yourselves these days, especially if you have your own strong dream of health and wellness to support it.

This isn't quite the idea of 'positive thinking' as such, as that idea somewhat implies 'staying positive in the midst of difficulty'. Although positive thinking has value, what is being said here is much more than that. This is strategically and rationally pointing ourselves in the direction of health and wellness, starting from the assumption that our brain is like a missile that can be fired in many different directions, and the key is to fire it in the direction we most want.

Of course, being told by the allopathic establishment that we only have a year to live will have the effect of pointing our brain in an unhelpful direction. It's a 'negative placebo', known as a 'nocebo'. That's not to say the establishment are 'wrong' about their diagnoses, and I understand they have to do their job, however, every prognosis is really a self-fulfilling prophesy. That's why it is important to be able to rebel. To say 'No' to the prognosis, and 'Yes' to Life. To say 'No' the illness and 'Yes' to wellness.

So just as it is important to pay attention to what we are feeding our bodies with, we have to begin to pay attention to what we are feeding our minds with. It's all very well being informed by educated and well-informed people, but if you are being fed negative placebos (nocebos), then it is worth noting the information being offered, but then quietly, gently and firmly choosing to align yourselves to outlooks that are more positive. In a sense, because we are all interrelated and interconnected, we are all constantly supporting each other in different ways with our thoughts, ideas and feelings, the question is…how am I supporting others and what is supporting me?

Linked to this, what is being discovered these days is the effect that the *quality* of our intention and thought has on our body and the world around us. More than thirty years ago, a Hawaiian doctor called Dr Len put into practice the principles of 'Ho'oponopono', which starts from the radical assumption that what is being observed is also being created by us. At the time he was working at the Hawaii state hospital on a ward for the criminally insane.

Over a period of time he sat in his office with the files of the patients and offered each one of them the words ''I love you, I'm sorry, Please forgive me, Thank you''. Little by little things began to change, shackles came off, the amount of drugs being administered went down, staff were happier to work there. Eventually prisoners started gradually to be released. After four years, the last couple of inmates were relocated somewhere else and the clinic for the mentally insane criminals was closed.

These days, the practice of Ho'oponopono is much more widely known and is recommended by many life coaches. Not only is it wonderful for our overall relationships, I highly recommend using it in regard to the illness. Sit quietly for a period each day, and with gently sincerity, offer the words 'I love you, I'm sorry, Please forgive me, Thank you' (the order of the statements can be changed). There are also musical recordings which can be played throughout the day or night which carry these words.

That is just one example of the power of intention, these days there are many. Dr Emoto conducted famous studies which suggested that if our intention is positive, and we are thinking loving thoughts about something, then it impacts very differently on what is being thought about as compared to thinking hateful thoughts. In one experiment, Dr Emoto placed portions of cooked rice into two containers. On one container he wrote "thank you" and on the other "you fool". He then instructed school children to say the labels on the jars out loud every-day when they passed them by. After thirty days, the rice in the container with positive thoughts was pretty much unchanged, while the other was mouldy and rotten! Given how much of the body is made up of water, he also thought it would be interesting to see the effect of positive intention on the structure of water crystals, and at least some of the studies showed a vast difference between water that was treated kindly and lovingly and water that was not.

There are also very interesting studies on meditation these days that not only show the positive impact of meditation on the brain, body and mind, but which also correlate the effect that it has on areas of the world that are in conflict or war. To offer just one example of many, a study of a two-month assembly in Israel during August and September of 1983 showed that, on days when the number of participants at a peace-creating assembly was high, the intensity of an ongoing war in neighbouring Lebanon decreased sharply. When the number of participants was high, war deaths in Lebanon dropped by 76 per cent!

The point is simply that our intention and quality of thought does have an effect. Which is really quite obvious when you think about it. In your family, or group of friends, when one is upset and angry, it has an effect on everyone else. It can be somewhat 'ignored', but we all know that a group dynamic in which everyone is happy and harmonious is better than a group dynamic in which someone is angry and unhappy.

Furthermore, it is now being argued and shown in a new branch of science called epigenetics, that the old view that DNA and genes controls our biology is a very incomplete picture of what's happening. Dr Bruce H. Lipton has shown that DNA is actually controlled by signals outside the cell, and that the energy that emanates from our thoughts is a powerful signal. As we retrain our thinking, and shift our focus, our bodies change! This new knowledge has the potential to bring an end to genetically passed on illness! It is also worth pointing out that the belief that 'illnesses are passed down genetically and there is nothing we can do' has actually been somewhat of a self-fulfilling prophecy itself (a nocebo), and is another example of how our beliefs have a way of self-justifying themselves.

Although positive feeling and intention is therefore very powerful, it's true that anger can be useful at times, in the sense that it is a wake-up call, a message to us that we are living below our standards, and it can help us to make changes and get out of bad situations. However, going to war with our bodies and hating the illness, or hating yourself for whatever reason, is not helpful, and neither is holding onto grievance and grudge.

A major reason for this is that, in our dreams of being healthy and well, we are not holding onto grievance and grudge. So bearing in mind that our brain takes direction from us, and doesn't place importance on the difference between reality and imagination, if we can be well in attitude, feeling and spirit NOW, then this is definitely going to be helpful. To put that another way, you may not be able to match the physical state that your body is in now to the physical state of your body in your dream, but you can match your state of *being* now, to the state of being in your dream.

So be committed to your exploration and focus but allow lightness to be here. Allow yourself as much as possible to enjoy the exploration. If it helps, laugh! Laughing is great for the body, mind and soul. Of course, what makes us laugh is a subjective thing, but sometimes there are things to laugh about in relation to the illness itself. My Mum's illness very much affected her movement, so that her walking was very stilted and juddering (not dissimilar to Parkinson's). I discovered that if I imitated her, it made her laugh! Not very politically correct perhaps, but still, laughing can definitely take weight and gravitas out of a situation, which is a healthy thing.

To be clear, I don't underestimate the challenge of doing this stuff, when you feel like crap. I may not have struggled with intense physical illness but I have experienced mental illness, and when things are bad, whether it is physical or mental, it can feel like being held at the bottom of a deep ocean with a cord around our legs, and we don't feel like we have the energy to do anything. Reaching for the light at the surface doesn't just feel like a challenge, it can seem impossible. On these occasions, reach for comfort, give yourself kindness, gentleness, peace, until conditions change just enough for you to be able to reach for something more dynamic. As a famous man once said, ''this too will pass'', and sometimes that is enough to get us through to the next day, when we can lift our head, raise our spirits and get focused on where we truly want to be.

The Challenge (Part One)

This isn't just about wanting to live, this is about being willing to be someone that completely overturns the prognosis, and this is a subtle but important difference. After all, most want to live, but not all will look outside of the conventional paradigm, and that's because convention can have a powerful hold over us. In a sense, we have to become someone that can stick two fingers up to the system! We have to be willing to be a bit of a leader or a pioneer.

So perhaps a bit strangely, the challenge is not *just* about finding what specifically is going to help us to recover, it is also about changing our focus, our attitude and our beliefs such that what CAN help us can show up for us. To be clear, this isn't hard for everyone by any means, some people are just keen to do what is necessary to get well, but human beings are complex and carry deep societal conditioning that can get in the way of taking new steps.

So here are some key principles or assumptions to work with. Even if they are not necessarily true, even if they over simplify the matter, they are a useful starting place (not dissimilar to the way that Ho'oponopono starts from the assumption that what we observe; we have created). These principles will give you a different way to look at your situation, they will shift your consciousness in such way that will enable you to perceive new and different ways forward.

1. It's not so much that an illness has been created and now you have to deal with it, health and

illness is an ongoing process that changes day by day.

2. There is nothing the body cannot recover from (rejuvenating limbs may be a bit of challenge, though I wouldn't rule anything out!). Your body is extremely intelligent and knows how to heal itself.
3. The illness is being created for a valid reason, it is not an accident, nor a punishment (though you might be creating illness as a way of punishing yourself for something).
4. We each play an active and participatory role in creating our states of health and illness.
5. The potential IS there to be well.
6. If you give the brain clear and consistent instruction, then it will lead the way.
7. A seeming miracle can happen, and can happen in an instant. The illness can literally be gone overnight (though if that's not how it is for you, then that's okay, it just means that you are interested in a different kind of path). It doesn't have to be arduous, it doesn't have to require effort, though you may be the kind that enjoys a good challenge!
8. It is good and often necessary to receive the support and assistance from others, and there are many experts out there waiting to help you, but ultimately, it is YOU that creates your health.

These principles may, to some extent, be in opposition to your understandings, then again, maybe your old understandings aren't serving you all that great at this point. Sometimes we have to be willing to put aside what seems 'true' or 'real', and instead, go with what *works*. Ultimately, if those principles turn out to be helpful, then you are really not going to care if they are true or not, you will be too busy enjoying your new life! And maybe this change in understandings is precisely the way in which you desire to grow at a deep level, and without the illness, you would never have been given the opportunity to look at things in a new way.

When we take on new principles and a new focus, we experience ourselves (and the world) differently, and this can be a sticking point. I will talk about this in terms of 'addiction' as it is very illustrative. A serious drug addict, that has been involved with...say....heroin for a number of years, is fully 'used' to who they are as a drug user. They are used to the particular sense of self that they have as someone that uses drugs. They are used to how their life feels, there is a deep familiarity with how they feel about themselves, even if they hate themselves and their life sucks. We all get comfort from the sense of familiarity with who we are, even if our lives as a whole are very uncomfortable. For the long term addict, it can be as hard letting go of that familiarity, as it is the chemical addiction itself. In the process of recovery, an addict will often face a seeming pit of inner emptiness that has them running back to the drug, even when rationally they know it's bad for them. The point is, that it's not *just* the drug that they are addicted to.

Finding comfort is how people survive deeply difficult conditions, whether it was in the concentration camps or being homeless on the street or in jail. As diabolical as the conditions are, as painful and uncomfortable as they are, there is a familiarity with our sense of 'who we are' (our sense of 'self') in that situation. Often we wonder how on earth people survive a certain situations, but we have the amazing capacity to find a level of comfort, it's part of being able to survive, and animals are the same.

The movie 'Shawshank Redemption' illustrated this very well. One of the prisoners had been in jail for most of his life, he was an old man by the time he was released on parole. He went out into the world theoretically a free man, but within a short space of time, he killed himself. When I first saw this I struggled to relate to why he would have done that, even though the movie did explain it well, it was only a few years later that I really began to 'get' it. Basically, the old guy had become fully used to his life on the inside, he was comfortable with it, he was comfortable with who he was, there was a deeply familiar sense of self, and he wasn't scared. On the outside, everything was unfamiliar including his sense of self, he lost all his sense of 'connection', and was scared all the time. As the movie explained, he had been 'institutionalized', he just couldn't cope with life on the outside.

This applies to illness and addiction too. We can become 'institutionalized' by our situation. We have to find a way to cope with the difficulty, and in the end we find a level of comfort in the familiarity, and who we are in relation to the illness/addiction. The idea of having a whole new focus, of changing the way we think and feel, of experiencing ourselves in a totally different way, can genuinely be intimidating. This is another reason why it is so important to have a strong celebratory dream of going dancing, or a dream of going to the Caribbean, or a dream of joyfully being at our grandchildren's wedding. The dream reminds us that it IS safe for us to be someone new, that we haven't ALWAYS been (and felt) ill, that there are other versions of ourselves that it is okay for us to be.

Anthony Robbins, the famous life coach, has also talked about this. He works with people while holding the assumption that the person's goal has to be more compelling than the prospect of things staying the same. If your goal isn't compelling, then make it so, or find one that it. As part of his approach, he invites people to imagine themselves in a year's time, in ten years' time, in thirty years' time in an unchanged situation. This has the effect of amplifying the discomfort of the current situation, and the compulsion to move away from that situation into something new and better is also amplified. In a sense, if you have been tolerating a bad situation for a long time, getting more uncomfortable with it can be a positive thing, but it is very important at the same time to having something positive to move towards.

He has also talked massively about the importance of focus. One great example he offered was when he had the opportunity to learn how to drive a racing car (Nascar I think). His instructor assured him that he would learn very quickly because the training car was set up so that people could learn quickly. Basically, the car had a switch which the instructor could push, which would make the car spin out off the road. The instructor told Tony that he HAD to keep his eye on the road when the car span, and the car would follow his focus. If he looked at the wall, the car would hit the wall. Tony started to drive and just as he got comfortable, the button was pushed and the car went into a spin. Initially he said that his eyes went to the wall, but the instructor yelled at him to look at the road, and he regained control at the last moment. This went on for several laps until Tony was conditioned to stay focused on the road, and he eventually went on to drive some very good laps.

This is how the process of getting well can unfold. There may be times when you spin out, when things seem terrible, when emotions are strong, when you feel like you have been beaten, but you have to get your eyes back on the road. You have to develop *resilience*. This is not an invitation to 'cope', which is a deeply negative idea (it assumes the worst), it is an invitation to pick yourself up, to remind yourself and feel the truth of your goal, and keep going. Persistence pays off.

Furthermore, if we have been struggling for many years, doing the same things and getting the same results, there can even be a level of embarrassment involved if we do something different and it gets a radically different result in a short space of time. We may look at ourselves and wonder why we didn't do it before! It can also be uncomfortable just being....wrong! If we have steadfastly believed in our prognosis for a number of years, if we have had conviction that the illness has nothing to do with us, if our view of society has been such that we have thought that the medical establishment knows best, if we have believed that there is nothing we can do.....it's not always easy to turn our world view on its head, and perhaps have to admit to ourselves (and others!) that we have been wrong.

Even with my understandings, it still often surprises me when those with a particular illness don't know about those that have recovered from their illness. I know a fair bit about Parkinson's because it was somewhat similar to my Mum's illness, and there are videos on YouTube that show that full recovery is possible. I recall one woman used Qigong (search in YouTube for "lilou mace Parkinson's") and another Australian chap by the name of John Coleman has said that meditation, flower essences and various kinds of bodywork were crucial to his recovery. But if I go to a major 'cure Parkinson's' website and search for his name, it doesn't even come up. It's very interesting. Putting aside conspiracy theories about pharmaceutical corporations, I would explain this by simply saying that the consensus focus of attention is not on those that recover, Perhaps also the popular cultural response is to see these kinds of recoveries as being for weirdy-beardies, wacky hippy types and new age tree huggers, but on closer inspection, these people are usually very grounded and very practical. What Western society often calls 'quackery', for other societies it is the norm. Countries such as Russia, China, India and Brazil have a LOT to offer in their approach to health.

So one of the reasons why old methods and beliefs stick around long after something better has come along is because it's not always easy letting go of the familiar, the comfortable, it's not easy being out there on the leading edge doing something different. Well, actually, it is for some people, some people are born leaders and pioneers, but many are not. I wouldn't say that I am a 'pioneer', but I do have an interest in what works, and it is because I am not 'naturally' a pioneer that I have an understanding of the challenges that many face in doing things differently. I have an understanding of the fears that many face in doing things differently.

The point is, the more willing you are to let go of old beliefs, and open your mind to new understandings, the better. Remember, we are shown what we believe most. So when we change our understandings, change our focus, different ways forward make themselves available.

Now, obviously a challenge is going to be finding what works for you, because even though one solution can work for many people, it may not be right for you. For example, with Cancer, some people swear by cannabis oil, others swear by baking soda, others swear by particular dietary changes. One example here:

http://www.mirror.co.uk/news/uk-news/man-cures-himself-of-cancer-using-1325900

(as an interesting point, note the slightly derogatory use of the word 'wacky')

Is this specific diet going to work for you? Perhaps, perhaps not.

Whether it's a 'wacky' diet, a supplement, a healing, or some kind of 'zapper', there is something for you out there, it may be a case of striking gold straight away, or there may be a process of exploration and following your intuition. There may well be disappointment and upset, there may be false starts. You have to keep the faith, you have to keep going, you have to stick to the dream. You may have people wonder what on earth you are doing, especially if there comes a point when you have to make a choice between conventional method and alternative method (choosing whether to receive chemotherapy or not is a classic difficult choice).

Another reason that conventional methods are stuck to, despite often very mixed results, is because we don't want to live with the shame of going against professional advice, and then failing. It's one thing to die having gone the chemotherapy route, it's another thing to die having stuck to a 'wacky' diet. We have to live by our choices. Twenty years ago, even ten years ago, the energy of support for making alternative choices was massively less than it is now. More and more, society as a whole is supporting and encouraging those that face the challenge of illness to find a path that works specifically for them.

There IS support for you these days in the choices you make.

The Challenge (Part 2).

As part of taking responsibility for our role in creating our state of health/illness, it can be extremely helpful to look at what we are getting out of the illness, and this is sometimes referred to as 'secondary benefits'. There can be a lot of resistance to doing this, we often don't like to think that we are getting *anything* out of the illness.

One of the main reasons that we can be resistant to this idea is because of the natural sympathy given by others for the pain and discomfort we experience. It's not that we feel we can't do without the sympathy, what we are not comfortable with is being given sympathy and attention, when there is also a background intuitive sense that we are getting something out of the illness, even if it is just the sympathy!! On some level we recognize that there is something slightly 'not quite right' about the dynamic, we probably don't want to actually reject the sympathy, so it becomes easier to say that the illness is a misfortune that is nothing to do with us, and that we couldn't possibly be getting something out of it. Point is, that offering sympathy or gravitating towards it, is not *always* a good thing.

In the case of Mum (for a couple of years I was the 'primary' caregiver), I noticed that she consistently responded in healthier ways to the world when I didn't give her a whole lot of sympathy for her situation. There were times when I did, when it was appropriate to console and tell her that I was sorry about her situation, but on a general day to day level, I didn't offer sympathy because I didn't want to make her feel like there was nothing she could do, and I also didn't want her to generate the kind of inner conflict that I described above.

I felt that to offer an excess of sympathy would have disempowered her, it would have programmed her with the belief that there was nothing she could do, that she was a victim of the illness. What I am saying here is somewhat counter-intuitive, and can perhaps *look* somewhat unfeeling at times, but love isn't always gooey and soft. It is important to remind ourselves sometimes that being given a compassionate hug feels nice, but how does it compare to the joy of swimming in the ocean, or witnessing our children give birth to their children?

Furthermore, an illness can be hugely painful and uncomfortable, but if we have been 'institutionalized' by it, then in a subtle way, it IS protecting us. We are getting a level of security out of it. Illness can also provide us with a challenge, something that we can really get our teeth stuck into, something that engages our attention. This may apply particularly to those whose children are grown up, and work life is over, and are feeling a bit 'lost'. Illness provides us with the potential to stretch ourselves and to grow. It can give us a sense of purpose. The idea of NOT having the illness may leave us wondering, ''what on earth would we do without it?!''. That's why you gotta have the dream. You have to have a powerful reason to be well.

Ironically, it is also often a fear of failure that stops us from taking radical steps. In one way, if we give our power to the illness and the doctors, then death is not our fault. However, if we take steps and fail, then we have to face the potential for failure. This is true for any innovator or anyone out there on the leading edge of change. It inevitably means facing failure at many points along the path. By equal measure, we are also scared of the success! We say, ''who am I to beat this illness when so many others have succumbed? Why should I be different? What makes me so special? What will I do with this new health…will I feel compelled to share what I did with others? Will I have to put myself forward in some way?''

Not only that, illness can provide us with connection to many people, both old and new. We can get friendly with our doctors, our social care visitors, we might attend particular support groups or join an online forum. We get to experience new aspects of the world through the illness even if we are confined in physical ways. Plus another hidden benefit is that our family tend to stay closer when we are ill. And of course, as much as we might say that we don't want to be pitied (and that's true), as humans we do like to be 'seen'. When we are ill, people naturally reach out to us and 'see' us. '

Sometimes, an illness can show up as a way of inviting us to change something in our lives. It might be a relationship, a job, a living environment. Or it might be asking us to look at our habits and our choices, it might be inviting us to look at our relationships with others and ourselves, or it might just be an invitation to re-prioritize our values. It may be that you genuinely need more attention and company in your life, in which case the illness is serving a purpose, so the challenge is to find ways to get attention and company that don't require you to be ill.

Equally, it might be inviting us to look at the way we handle emotion/feeling (for example, perhaps we bottle up anger), or it might be a prompt to resolve an issue from the past that may not seem remotely relevant to who we are today. Many that experience abuse of different kinds when they are young grow up with emotional scars, but don't recognize that the wound may still be playing itself out in our lives. An illness can be a trigger to look at that.

Brandon Bays in her book 'The Journey' describes her recovery from an enormous tumour, it was indeed a 'journey' with successes and disappointments, but which ended with full recovery, and in her own words, she ''uncovered a means to get direct access to the boundless healing potential inside us all''. She has created a step by step process that reveals emotional memories and patterns stored in the cells that can be resolved and cleared so that the body can naturally and easily heal itself. Her method has been used for physical and emotional issues of many kinds and gets great results.

Lester Levenson's story is also very interesting. From www.sedona.com

''Lester Levenson was a man who had mastered life's greatest challenge. In 1952, at age 42, Lester, a physicist and successful entrepreneur, was at the pinnacle of worldly success, yet he was an unhappy, very unhealthy man. He had many health problems including depression, an enlarged liver, kidney stones, spleen trouble, hyperacidity, and ulcers that had perforated his stomach and formed lesions. He was so unhealthy, in fact, that after having his second coronary, his doctors sent him home to his Central Park South penthouse apartment in New York City to die.

Lester was a man who loved challenges. So, instead of giving up, he decided to go back to the lab within himself and find some answers. Because of his determination and concentration, he was able to cut through his conscious mind to find what he needed. What he found was the ultimate tool for personal growth—a way of letting go of all inner limitations. He was so excited by his discovery that he used it intensively for a period of three months. By the end of that period, his body became totally healthy again. Furthermore, he entered a state of profound peace that never left him through the day he died on January 18, 1994.''

Following this. Lester developed a technique called, 'The Sedona Method', and it is a very powerful method of 'releasing'. I am not suggesting that you rush out to get involved in this (or in anything else I am suggesting). the purpose is more to illustrate that there IS a lot of great stuff out there, that there ARE many that support the process of getting well, and that there IS hope.

As part of looking into the illness, it can also be helpful to notice what was going on with you and around you when the illness started. Did it start around the time you got a new job? Or moved house? Or when a relationship went sour? Or when you started to wonder what to do with your life? These are just examples.

Depending on your illness, it is also worthwhile noticing specifically when symptoms show up and when there is respite. In some cases this doesn't apply obviously, but in the case of many conditions and disorders....whether its digestion issues, heart issues, mental health issues such as schizophrenia, nervous system issues, or autism, the difficulties are not wholly consistent. There is variance. There is a level of subjectivity. There are *clues.*

My Mum's illness was fascinating in that way. She was diagnosed with 'Progressive Supranuclear Palsy' (it's worth noting that when an illness is actually *titled* as 'progressive', a very powerful nocebo is created!), but in the end I came to think in terms of *when* she PSP-ed and when she didn't. In a sense, it became a verb rather than a noun. For example I noticed that she PSP-ed most when feeling self-conscious. When do you Parkinson's? When do you MS? Is it when you are stressed? When you are feeling under pressure? Is it when you are doing something you don't want to do? Is it when you are tired or frustrated? Is it when you sit in a particular chair, or haven't had fresh air in a while? Is it spend time with certain people?

In the case of my Mum, after a while, I was able to predict with great accuracy as to when she would struggle and when she was at ease. In the comfort of the lounge with no sense of being pressured, she could stand on her feet for long periods, probably indefinitely. If she was out in public and feeling self-conscious. .over she would go with unerring consistency. Frustration was another key factor for her, especially if she was angry with herself or her body, not only would she lose her balance, but she would consistently somehow find a way to bang her head on something sharp and dangerous. It had 'punishment'' written all over it.

To give another example, when she was under pressure, she struggled to speak. The more effort she put in, the less she was able to. My Mum came from a world in which she was very much conditioned to speak with great politeness, and perhaps oddly, this was also a factor in the symptoms. When she was carrying an image of politeness, she struggled to talk. When she had something she needed to say directly from the heart, from her being, she was able to speak with more ease.

These are the kinds of things I'm talking about. Get interested in your illness - when it shows up, when it recedes. In the case of Mum and probably many similar situations, meditation was good for her, exercise was good for her (it connected her very directly to her body), and physical body work was great for her, whether it was yoga or massage. It's all good. Furthermore, if you can, get interested in the nature of health and illness itself, get interested in the science of success, get interested in the relationship between the body and mind.

The whole process of becoming aware in this way can require us to drop a level of pride. We may have thought that an illness is nothing to do with us, that it is a random affliction from a cruel world or an unjust God, but it's far more helpful to notice the way in which we are involved in the illness. That's not an invitation to blame ourselves, it's an invitation to take an empowered approach. To begin to notice, without judgement, the characteristics of the illness. You may even find that watching certain kinds of movies or listening to certain kinds of music are not beneficial.

As you notice these things, be willing to change your habits. Quite often we fatally (quite literally) hear someone say that 'the illness won't change me'....or post mortem we might hear someone say with fondness, ''the illness never changed him/her''. I'm sorry if this sound rude, but 'forget' that! Seriously. Allow yourself to change! The illness is being created for a reason, and if health requires you to respond to the world in a new way, to change the way you relate to the world, to get some new habits and interests, then get going with that. Determination and 'will' is a wonderful thing, but stubbornness is not. Love yourself and your family enough to change if necessary. Be determined, but flexible.

The confusion about 'whether an illness should change us or not' is a slight misunderstanding about who we are. Ultimately, our true and indefinable individualness is present with OR without the illness. At the deepest level, the illness doesn't change us, but then neither does recovery. These are all just experiences you are having, they are explorations of life. Allow yourself to be different in the world if that is what it means to be well, be different in your relationships if that is what it means to be well, but know that who you are is much more than *what's happening,* either with, or without an illness. The illness MAY even be an invitation to realize that who/what you are is prior to anything that happens.

I recently watched a video of a Mother and her daughter, the Mother has Alzheimer's. She awoke from the illness for a while and recognized her daughter and the scene that followed was very moving and they told each other that they loved each other. The wonderful thing about humanity is that our love is deeper and goes beyond 'what's happening'. The daughter doesn't stop loving her Mum just because her personality has changed and she doesn't recognize her. I would argue that Mum also doesn't stop loving her daughter, even though the personality aspect is such that she doesn't recognize her. In those moments in which Mum is present, it is clear that the love remains untouched. We love each other despite personality changes, despite life choices, despite our habits. We may not choose to spend time with our loved ones if there are changes, and that's fine, but the love itself doesn't change, it is in fact, eternal.

As an aside, I am no expert on Alzheimer's or similar kinds of conditions, but it seems to me that 'being present' is very important. Obviously there comes a point when this is irrelevant, but in the early stages, or preferably well before, doing something like meditation might be very helpful. There are some great brain training websites online which I suspect are also very good for us.

The main points here are, firstly, that health (and illness) is not something you *have* as much as it is something that you create as an ongoing process. You can be creating health one minute and creating illness the next. Someone who is consistently healthy knows how to create health for themselves consistently. Any moment in which your symptoms are not present is a moment of health. So it's not so much that someone *has* good health, it's more that someone has the awareness of how to create consistent health for themselves, whatever that looks like. To be clear, for some that might mean a meat diet, for others it might mean a veggie diet. For some it might mean strong exercise, for others it might be relaxing more. For some it might mean having more fun, for others it might mean living with more purpose.

Secondly, it is important to be open and willing to change your 'personality self'. Be open and willing to feel different, to experience yourself differently, to recognize yourself differently, to drop what is associated with illness. Even though we can definitely get comfortable with our sense of self during illness, and it very much SEEMS like we are 'being ourselves' when we are ill, it's probably more true that when you experience yourself as well and vibrant that you are a more accurate reflection of who you are at the deepest level. Sometimes this might mean being willing to sacrifice our sense of self as an ill person in order to become a well person, a person that overturns the prognosis. I am reminded of Richard Bandler, a very powerful facilitator of change, who once said, 'why be yourself, when you can be someone so much better?' This can be a very good question to ask ourselves at times.

****

Now if this all sounds like hard work…..well, it can be. But it doesn't HAVE to be. It really might just be as simple as putting the book down, reading something on the internet, having a go at it….and hey presto! It can be extremely straight forward, it really doesn't have to require much change, but I want to cover the bases here in the book, and I know that sometimes illness can be very 'sticky', and sometimes, we are the glue itself keeping us stuck to it.

Illness may seem like a battle with the body, but ultimately it a psychological battle that is won and lost in the mind. It took me a long time to get that. It is of course massively helpful to address bodily symptoms in the myriad of ways that can be done, and undoubtedly, addressing the body will also affect the mind. In this sense, they are not separate. Work on the mind, and the body will change, equally, work on the body and the mind will change. Give your brain consistent clear instruction and things will start to unfold in a positive direction for you.

I also want to be clear that this isn't about 'doing everything you can' so that you can say just before you die that 'you did everything you could'. Martyrdom is no use here, and neither is victimhood. It's entirely possible to take action towards getting well, without really meaning it, or secretly believing that it's futile, or doing it for the sake of others. This is very different from persistently doing what it takes to be healthy and well.

Similarly, it's not quite about doing what it takes to 'beat the illness', because the illness is not some alien enemy outside of you, it is a bunch of symptoms that the body is creating for whatever reason it is doing so. We can say that we hate the illness, that we would never want such a thing, that we would never choose such a thing…..and certainly we may experience hating the illness and not wanting the illness, but there is another truth here as well, one that is often hard to admit to ourselves. It is very helpful to get radically self-honest here, to take a look and say…..''Hmmm. Okay. On some level, I am involved in choosing this situation''. This is not an invitation to feel bad, to feel ashamed, to feel scared, it's an invitation to take responsibility for your state, and then do what it takes.

To be clear, if all this sounds like too much, that's really okay too. Sometimes it is more appropriate just to fully allow what's unfolding to unfold. Sometimes the key lesson and growth IS the allowing, it IS the peace, it IS the making the most of the tail end of your life. I'm not saying you *should* be well, I truly understand that sometimes we are ready to transition to a whole new dimension, we are ready for heaven. I truly understand that sometimes, the highest service we can offer to our loved ones and to the world is to allow ourselves to pass. Death is not a mistake nor an accident, and the more consciously it is chosen, the more peace there will be in the transition. I'm not advocating Life here because I think death is something to be scared of, I think life after death is probably a whole lot easier than life on earth! I can see the appeal! I am advocating Life here because I think it's wrong that people DON'T feel they have a choice, that people are lead to believe that they are powerless, that people feel obliged to play out the prophecies and negative placebos that they are given by good-intentioned doctors. I believe the system is currently flawed, and it doesn't have to be that way. If you want to live, there *are* steps for you to take.

Proactive Steps

It doesn't matter what your religious and spiritual leanings are (or absence thereof), it is worth considering the power of 'prayer'. My guess is that serious illness often has a way of inviting us to question our beliefs about life and God, and even those that wouldn't normally say a prayer, might be drawn to consider the idea. We all know there are millions of prayers 'sent' to God every day, and the evidence often suggests that they don't do any good. I would suggest that all prayers are answered, if not by God, then by Life itself, but the way they are answered is determined by the kind of prayer that we engage in.

As I said earlier, what we focus on we get more of. If we send out a prayer full of lack and poverty, then the answer to our prayer is likely to take the form of more lack and poverty. Equally, asking for the strength to 'cope', is likely to only give us more difficult situations to 'cope' with!

A positive prayer that comes with gratitude and abundance is far more effective. Specifically thanking God (or whatever name your 'God' goes by) for your current experience, asking God show you the way to health and happiness, and then thanking God for that positive outcome, can be a powerful thing.

Here is what Neale Donald Walsch usefully has to say on the subject, ''Gratitude in advance is the most powerful creative force in the universe. Most people do not know this, yet it is true. Expressing thankfulness in advance is the way of all Masters. So do not wait for a thing to happen and then give thanks. Give thanks before it happens, and watch energies swirl! To thank God before something occurs is an act of extraordinary faith. And that, of course, is where the power comes from.''.

There doesn't have to be a prayer every morning or every day. A single sincere prayer may be enough. Please consider this as an option even if you are agnostic. Personally, I have no problem with the idea of 'God' but if it helps it doesn't even really matter if there is a 'God' or not, what is important is that a powerful message is put out there to Life, one that your body and brain also clearly hears. There is a bit of a science and an art to prayer, and if you need help with it, there are some great prayers on YouTube. While you are there, search for 'Thomas Fischer', a street healer. The strong religious tone may put some off, but the methodology behind the healings is very interesting and clearly has a potent effect. This same methodology can be applied in less religious verbiage, in the end, the way we 'code' these things is far less important than the result.

On a similar theme, the 'law of attraction' is often talked about these days in spiritual and personal development arenas, and this is well worth investigating. 'The Secret' is probably the most well-known law of attraction book/film, but there are many teachers, and perhaps 'Abraham-Hicks' is the most popular.

In a nutshell, it is the idea that when our state of being/mind is a 'vibrational match' to our desire, then what we desire has to show up. To put that another way, our circumstances (including the circumstance of our body-mind) reflect our state of being. If we feel well, then we will attract to us circumstances that reflect wellness. Similarly if we are focused upon an absence of wellness, then our circumstances mirror that too.

While I would say that talking about the circumstances of our life ONLY in terms of the 'law of attraction' is an oversimplification, and somewhat ignores many factors at play, it is definitely a useful principle to understand, and some of the exercises that trail in its wake are very powerful. Bearing in mind that if you feel good now, then the universe will reflect that back at you, you might (for example) want to sit and write a pretend (but authentic) letter to a friend or relative from a place of having recovered from the illness. Talk about how good you feel, all the wonderful things you are doing, how easy and effortless your body is functioning. You get the idea. This is just one example of many practices that you could do, again, YouTube has a huge amount of videos on the subject, and there are many law of attraction forums too.

Here is one more popular process that is designed to shift your state of mind, state of being and overall state of health. It is an Abraham-Hicks process and is called 'Reclaiming One's Natural State of Health Process.' Do this process while lying in a comfortable place. Choose a time when you have approximately fifteen minutes when you are not likely to be disturbed. Have this list ready for you to read, and when you first lie down, read it slowly to yourself.....

It is natural for my body to be well.

Even if I don't know what to do in order to get better, my body does.

I have trillions of cells with individual Consciousness, and they know how to achieve their individual balance.

When this condition began, I didn't know what I know now.

If I had known then what I know now, this condition couldn't have gotten started.

I don't need to understand the cause of this illness.

I don't need to explain how it is that I'm experiencing this illness.

I have only to gently, eventually, release this illness.

It doesn't matter that it got started, because it's reversing its course right now.

It's natural that it would take some time for my body to begin to align to my improved thoughts of Well-Being.

There's no hurry about any of this.

My body knows what to do.

Well-Being is natural to me.

My Inner Being is intricately aware of my physical body.

My cells are asking for what they need in order to thrive, and Source Energy is answering those requests.

I'm in very good hands.

I will relax now, to allow communication between my body and my Source.

My only work is to relax and breathe.

I can do that.

I can do that easily.

After finishing the list, continue to relax, focus on your breathing and allow the feeling of well-being to be here. Be as comfortable as possible without forcing it. You will likely feel soft, gentle sensations in your body, this is healing energy specifically answering your cellular request. Do nothing to try to help it, just continue to relax, breathe. allow and enjoy it.

****

I would also strongly recommend getting a 'vision board' or plastering your walls with pictures that inspire you and make you feel good. Not just a few, LOTS. For example, on google images you could put in 'dancing on the beach' and then 'print' what appeals to you. You want to be able to wake up in the morning and see these pictures, remember, the brain doesn't care what is imagined and what is real, just looking at them will give your brain the right message, and will do your state of being the world of good. If, like me, you lean towards spirituality, you could also print off pictures of the angels and masters and put them on your walls, they are also great for our energy. It's also good to have plenty of plant life in your house, plants have a way of connecting us to the power of life.

The importance of having a dream has already been talked about, but Dr David Hamilton has illustrated just how powerful visualization and imagery can be. In his own words, ''the key here is to create an internal image (you don't need to be a good visualizer and see in HD.

We all imagine in our own ways) of the conditions. Ten people will come up with ten different images so there's not actually a right or wrong way to do it. It's an image or set of images that feel true for you, perhaps based on how you feel, intuition, or a description that a medical person has given you. This is your picture of 'illness'. Then you convert it in your imagination to a picture of 'wellness'. The secret is simply changing from illness into wellness. You can do it in any way you want, using tools, energy, light, just imagining forms changing....whatever you want, really, so long as you convert illness into wellness. And you do it over and over and over again, like every day, preferably a couple of times a day.''

David's book, ''How the Mind Can Heal the Body'' is excellent, and within it are actual examples of people that used imagery to recover from their condition. Even if you are not someone that can easily do this kind of thing (I am also not), it is still powerful reading.

You also might want to consider getting some 'subliminal messages' that you can play in the background during the day or at night while you sleep. There are some that relate specifically to health which would obviously be useful, but one in particular that I always thought was powerful was on the subject of 'miracles'. Many of us have been conditioned to believe that seemingly miraculous change is impossible, and it's not. We have also been taught that radical change has to take time, and even this is not necessarily true. You might find that change comes very quickly for you, or you may find that after a period in which nothing much has changed, that doors suddenly start to open up for you. Sometimes it takes a period of time to prepare us for rapid change. Hypnotherapy is also very good, if you went to see a hypnotherapist in person that would be great, but there are also many cheap, good, downloads available these days. Again, these can be put on at night when you go to bed.

I also strongly recommend getting some 'energy' support, in the many different forms in which it comes. Reiki is the most well-known, and is a very benevolent and supportive energy, it definitely wouldn't hurt to ask someone to send you Reiki every week. On the internet these days, there are Reiki practitioners that will offer their services very cheaply, often free. You could also look on www.fiverr.com where you will find many healers of different kinds, all of which will send you Reiki for a 'fiver'. Qigong is also a very strong and supportive energy, and there are again many that would be happy to send you energy. On this website, you can sign up to receive free energy support in the form of Qigong http://www.qigongenergyhealing.com/ but there are many others. Reconnective healing tends to be a bit more expensive, but can be VERY powerful. It suggests that three sessions are best, and I would trust that. As with all the others, Reconnective energy can be sent from a distance, but in this instance I would recommend going to see someone in person, it's not as popular as Reiki, but there are still practitioners everywhere. Then there is Quantum Touch Healing which I have no personal experience of, but understand it is very good. In the UK, in most decent sized towns, spiritual healers tend to offer their services once a week on a donation basis, and again, this can very useful support.

Then there are more 'specialist' type healings which can be excellent. There are so many good healers out there that I wouldn't suggest paying much for a healing, and personally, I question any healer that is charging huge amounts of money. A great modality that I definitely recommend is called 'Spiritual Response Therapy', the practitioners use their skills to take a really close look at what's going on with your illness and will clear any issues around it. NSR energy healings are also excellent, though my opinion is that they are at the border in terms of the price that I consider to be reasonable (your border may well be different). Bio-Energy Balancing is also very much worth looking at, shamanic healings can be good, past life healings, Melchizadek Method.....there is so MUCH out there these days, I am not even scratching the surface here. If you are interested I suggest exploring for yourself, though I will say again that Spiritual Response Therapy is a somewhat 'grounded' option for those that are not spiritually inclined, and can often get to the root of issues.

Then there are the less 'spiritually inclined' modalities, many of which you will be familiar with, but all have value and can make profound differences in some cases. Acupuncture, Bowen Technique, Craniosacral Therapy, Reflexology are all excellent, please have a look at them. There is also a modality called BodyTalk which I do have a fair bit of experience with and I highly recommend: http://www.bodytalkuk.co.uk/ This modality has the ability to look at all your sensitivities and intolerances, it is able to see if there has been any poisoning, or fungus, or parasites, and it can clear them all from your body. There are practitioners at 'fiverr' that are offering this modality from a distance, and they are great, but they are not as comprehensive as an 'in person' appointment.

Any issue that comes with 'physical' challenges is likely to benefit from some kind of activity like yoga, Pilates or Alexander Technique. Then there is Oxygen Therapy, which can be pricy, but is reportedly very good for some conditions such as cancer, strokes, heart disease and even Aids. It doesn't come cheap, but it is possible to rent out a machine on a month by month basis which could work out much better. It requires only twenty minutes a day. One to investigate I feel.

The world of 'supplements' is a minefield, but one worth exploring. There are many famous ones like fish oil and probiotics (great for Crohn's), but the key obviously is to look at what has been working for others, and this requires research, but a single supplement can make a massive difference to arthritis, blood pressure, autism, Parkinson's and many more. When I used to spend time on the forum that was relevant to Mum's illness (PSP), I noticed there was a caregiver there giving her Dad lots of particular supplements, and she was reporting a definite improvement in many different ways. It was very encouraging to see, though not applicable to Mum because of her difficulties with swallowing at the time. Nevertheless, there are people out there making a difference by using supplements. Equally, juicing is now known for its potent effects, and even just a simple thing like adjusting our acid/alkaline ratio can facilitate amazing body-mind changes.

Less well known is the potential problem of 'geopathic stress' (and also electromagnetic stress), which is linked to earth vibrations and the electromagnetic field. There is a huge amount of information online, just one example I pulled off the top of a google search is this: http://www.rolfgordon.co.uk/ It seems that it can be a factor in a very wide range of issues from Cancer to M.E to Autism to Bipolar Disorder to difficulties with conceiving. There are effective, but expensive, devices which balance out the issue, but it can also be resolved more cheaply here: http://www.intelligentenergies.com (again just one example). This is the kind of thing that I would recommend doing because at a bare minimum, it's not going to hurt, and at best, it might be something that makes a big difference to certain conditions.

A couple of times I have mentioned the 'zapper', and here is a link: http://www.drclark.net

A heavy metal detox might be useful:
http://www.howtodetoxheavymetals.com/

One link of many to the benefits of cannabis oil:
http://www.dailymail.co.uk/health/article-2725748/Cannabis-oil-helped-cured-cancer-claims-father-given-two-years-live.html

The benefits of coconut oil in relation to Alzheimer's (and this is one of MANY stories of full recovery):
http://healthimpactnews.com/2013/film-to-be-made-of-fathers-recovery-from-alzheimers-with-coconut-oil/

And here is some good news for those with MS:
http://www.overcomingmultiplesclerosis.org/Recovery-Program/Program-Overview/

And much to be positive about here:
http://www.alswinners.com/

The final thing that I want to talk about here (and it's not final because it's the only thing left to say, there is SO much that could be said in this section), is EFT, and Faster EFT.

EFT is short for Emotional Freedom Technique, and it involves tapping on various parts of our body. It looks a bit strange, and if you are not used to doing this kind of self-help malarkey, then you might feel a bit foolish initially, but the results speak for themselves. So many people have resolved emotional, mental and physical issues using EFT. It might be particularly relevant for those with symptoms that respond to stress, for example Crohn's, or Parkinson's or M.S, but there are many other potential issues that EFT could have bearing on. On YouTube, Brad Yates is very popular, and keeps it simple, but I would highly recommend working with someone in your area if you can, as a personal practitioner can work with your specific issue.

There is also a new version called Faster EFT, which mixes EFT with neuro-linguistic programming. Originated by Robert Smith, I have only experienced this on YouTube, but the results that people get in relation to all sorts of different conditions, are excellent. If there is someone in your area, again, might well be worth considering.

****

I think that's enough proactive steps to offer, the saying goes 'enough is as good as a feast', and I think that applies here. The intention here is really just to give you some ideas and get you started. I don't want to create an over-whelm. However, if you want any more personal recommendations or support of some kind (bearing in mind I am not a qualified expert) my contact will be at the back of the book, please get in touch, anything I offer would be free.

Conclusion

I want to be clear again that none of this is about *avoiding death* as such, which self-evidently has its place in our lives and is entirely natural. There is a time to transition, a time that is right for each soul, and that's all well and good. What this is book is about, is choice. It's about recognizing that you are never helpless, never powerless, never without options, and if it's not right for you to take proactive steps towards health, then that is a valid choice. This might reflect an intuitive sense that maybe you have done all that you needed to do, experienced all that you needed to experience, and that maybe all that's left is to embrace your path joyfully towards the next chapter beyond this life. Equally though, it might suggest that relaxing is the most important thing that you can do for yourself at this particular point in your path, and that even though taking steps is not appropriate for you in this moment, that might well change for you sometime soon. Be open to change, even if it's not right for you at this moment.

So I am not saying you *should* take steps, or that it is necessarily the best thing for you to take steps. Nevertheless, it is important for me to show that, contrary to what you might have been told, or currently believe, that there *are* potential steps that can be taken, that there is a new way of thinking about your illness, that there are certain principles that can be usefully applied. It has also been necessary to show you what might be blocking you from moving forward, and to give you some practical suggestions as to what might be good for you.

I didn't want this to be a long book, I wanted it to be short, and if not sweet, then at least a bit 'potent', in that I would like you to close this page with a slightly new way of seeing the world, and a slightly new 'consciousness'. It is my belief that every illness has its own 'energy', or its own 'consciousness', and this is created historically by all of us. For example, as a global collective, we have created cancer, and we all also the potential to create health. Although my Mum didn't recover from PSP, she far outlived the prognosis, and perhaps even more importantly, she was exercising and spending time with friends the day before she transitioned! There was no hospice, no massive drama, no major suffering. I believe that the work she did would have done something to change the energy and consciousness of that condition.

My point is, that even if you do nothing at all after reading this, perhaps just taking on some of the ideas, taking on the energy of hope, will have done something to change the condition that many others struggle with. Equally, if you are a carer, please know that your positive attitude isn't just helping your loved one, but is making a difference on a much broader scale. Whether you are the one with a condition, or a carer, thank you for doing your bit.

It is important that you have positive people in your life. Kind people with good intentions may be offering you plenty of understanding and sympathy, but you need people that aren't perpetuating nocebos, people that can hold a positive vision for you. If there is no-one like that in your close circle, get yourself onto a forum of some kind, or go find a holistic doctor that will see your future in a positive way. Join groups that will give you positive placebos. If you can afford it, go to an Anthony Robbins seminar and walk across fire! Find an EFT Practitioner in your area. Get yourself a good massage or reflexology therapist. Join a yoga class. Fill your house with pictures and plants that rejuvenate your spirit. Be good to yourself, kind to yourself, hold your dream, and be persistent. There are MANY people doing this these days, and this is a movement that is far more grounded and realistic than is sometimes thought, I come from a very 'normal' background myself. Many extremely intelligent scientists are exploring and writing on these subjects these days, and I feel it won't be long before we are witnessing a revolutionary convergence between allopathic and 'alternative' medicine. Allow yourself to be involved in this change,

As Ghandi said, "Be the change you wish to see in the world." It is my belief that we all wish to see and experience a world free from disease of any kind, and together we are creating this new reality. Here, the idea of 'the hundredth monkey effect' seems relevant. For those that aren't familiar with it, it is rooted in the account of some unidentified scientists that were conducting a study of macaque monkeys on the Japanese island of Koshima in 1952. These scientists observed that some of these monkeys learned to wash sweet potatoes, and slowly this new behaviour spread through the younger generation of monkey. There finally came a point, the 'hundredth monkey' that this previously learned behaviour instantly spread across the water to monkeys on nearby islands. In a sense, the new behaviour was 'transmitted through consciousness' across the species at a certain point.

Whether this story is true or not, it usefully describes a 'tipping point', in which slow change suddenly becomes a quantum leap. I believe that we are at that tipping point, and that you are integral to that tipping point. What you are choosing to experience might well be looked back on as an amazing thing, and crucial to a revolution in health and wellness. You could be that hundredth monkey! :)

Blessings,

Andrew.

Please find me at <u>fumblingthroughthelight@gmail.com</u> or on Facebook at 'fumbling through the light', or our blog, fumblingthroughthelight.blogspot.co.uk